Dedication

This book is dedicated to every child living with sickle cell disease. We are all true warriors! To my mother, who worked tirelessly with me to make this book a reality, I appreciate you more than you know. Thanks for the love, encouragement, support and for keeping me grounded.

Contents

Contents iv
Welcome to My World 1
What It's Like to Be Me 4
Why My Diet is Important 11
School Life 18
What Happens When I Get Sick? 22
My Dreams and Fears 31
When I Grow Up 36

Welcome to My World!

My name is Alexia. I live in Texas. I am eight years old. I am an only child. I wish I had sisters and brothers... well maybe just a sister. Boys are sometimes annoying. My best friend is Natalie. She has a little brother, Nathan. I love dolls and teddy bears. Mom said I needed to get a job to support my doll and bear shopping habits. I started an e-commerce business. It is going well so far. My absolute favorite toys are my puppets. I have 8 of them. Their names are Roger, Stephanie, Olivia, Jack, Vanessa, Vincent, Bobby and Lexi. I have had them since I was two years old. That makes them six-years old. I love to go 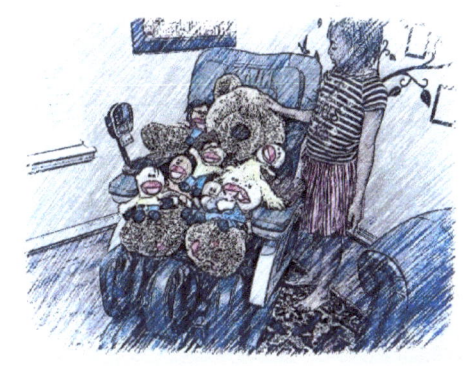 on imaginary trips with my puppets to places I can only dream of. Mom says I can always escape boredom in my imagination. In my imagination, the puppets each has a personality and can converse with each other. Sometimes we go to Paris, Italy, Spain, Holland and Scotland.

Another reason my puppets are special to me is, when I was almost three years old, I had difficulty expressing myself. My mother used these puppets to help me. I used to think they could speak. I would talk to the puppets all the time. As I grew older, I realized my mother was talking through the puppets like a ventriloquist. Whenever I got sick, only the puppets could cheer me up. I have sickle cell disease. Maybe you have heard of it before. If you haven't, it is when your red blood cells are abnormal and shape like a crescent or sickle. Red blood cells transport oxygen though the body. When they are sickled, they are not able to do that job so well. They also die much faster than regular red blood cells. As a result, there is not enough of them in the body at any given time. This causes anemia. Anemia makes me feel tired. Sometimes, I get dehydrated and then red blood cells stick together. They can't flow through the blood vessels smoothly enough in that state. It hurts. That is called a pain crisis. There are other complications associated with sickle cell disease, like pneumonia, asthma, acute chest syndrome, stroke, to name a few. My puppet, Lexi, has sickle cell disease too.

Sometimes, my mom plays with me. She is not crazy about dolls, except for Emma and Emily. Emma and Emily are life-sized dolls and it is easier to dress them. Mom thinks barbie dolls are too skinny and their clothes too tight. Personally, I think her fingers are too big. Other times, she takes me to the park, Adventure Kids or Monkey Joes for a play date. Overall, I have a good life.

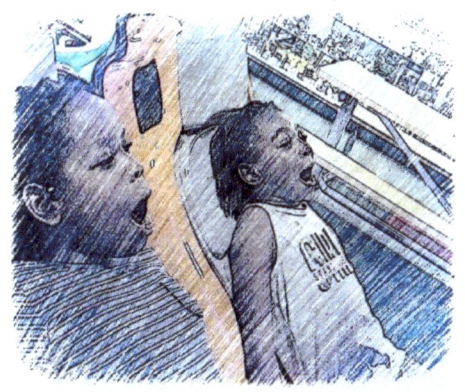

What It's Like to Be Me!

I am like any other eight-year-old. I love to play. I have lots of friends. I go to church. I love to hang out with my mom. I sing. I dance. I play the piano. I love spending time with Natalie. We do all kinds of girl things. Natalie plays the piano too. But there are some things I must do differently because of sickle cell. The main thing is that I must drink a ton of water, especially on hot days. Staying hydrated is super important. Why? Dehydration causes the blood to be thicker. The sickled red blood cells clump together resulting in pain crises. In my house, the options for staying hydrated are plain purified water or coconut water. I am not a big fan of coconut water. But once, I was in the pool for a long time and forgot to drink enough water. I was extremely dehydrated. My mom gave me coconut water. Ugh! Mom said dehydration results from potassium loss. Since coconut water is rich in potassium, it is a good option to rehydrate. Man! Why can't I just have some

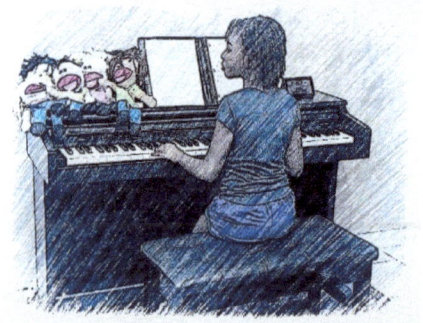

Gatorade like everybody else? Mom says because the dangers outweigh benefits. Gatorade is loaded with artificial colors and high levels of processed sugar. These increase health risks. Besides, Gatorade was designed for serious athletes, whose strenuous routines allow then to burn off the extra sugar. That does not describe me! That was the last time I neglected to drink enough water. I'll reserve the coconut water for extreme cases only.

  Now, let's talk about food. There are rules I must abide by. My mom supports a democracy. But when it comes to what I eat, she is not one. Eating pre and probiotic rich food is mandatory in my house. That took some getting used to. Mom says food is medicine. It is not just for pleasure. So, the first rule of eating in my house is knowing what is in your food. Mom taught me how to read food labels and to know when it is ok to eat it and when it isn't. This knowledge comes in handy when my friends try to share their snacks with me. For example, one day a friend offered me some apple juice. One 8-ounce serving had 28 grams of sugar. Now, 8 oz is not a lot of juice. Drinking the equivalent of 7 teaspoons of sugar in 8 ounces of apple juice is not a wise choice. That is more than the daily recommended amount of sugar in only 8 ounces of fluid. My mom never buys fruit juice. We keep processed food to a minimum. Once in a blue moon I get a single doughnut from the bakery section of the grocery store. Those moments are rare. So, it makes it that much more special. After all, I am still a kid! My mom may be optimistic, but she is still realistic. I wasn't always this good about watching what I eat. I'll tell you about that later.

    The great thing is that when my mom knows I will be with my friends, she comes up with a healthier version of food kids love to eat. She makes cookies with a gluten-free oat flour and a little maple syrup instead of sugar. She adds flavor-enhancing baking oils to make up for the lack of sugar. She makes doughnuts, beignets, oatmeal chocolate chip cookies, oatmeal raisin cookies... orange cranberry, lemon blueberry, cranberry walnut... banana nut muffins, double chocolate muffins, lemon-raspberry muffins... The double chocolate banana muffin is my favorite. My friends love my mom's cookies.

    We mainly eat at home. We pack food when we are traveling. That Yeti cooler can keep things cold for days, even in the summer. We even have a car microwave. Mom makes pancakes and waffles at home from scratch with coconut or almond flour. They are so good. The kids at school get excited whenever my mom comes to school. Even the teachers and parents look forward to eating her meals. My teacher says that after a while of eating my mom's food, she loses appetite for junk food and she doesn't crave sugar so much. I have eaten at McDonald's three times in my life while I was visiting relatives out of town. My mom was not at all happy when I told her. I don't understand the craze anyway. It tastes weird.

It used to bug me is that I am not allowed to eat candy. I didn't think that was fair. My friends get to eat it all day long. I used to take candy from my friends. But every time I did, my mom knew. I think she has eyes in the back of her head and hidden cameras in the house. I searched my backpack to see if there was one hidden there too. She even found the candy I hid in my closet. Mom spoke to my teacher about it. The kids were told not to share candies with me. That was the end of that. What was the big deal? It was only candy! The other parents bought candy for their kids. Why couldn't I have it? Mom explained to me that she knew for a while I was taking candy from my friends. She was not opposed to the occasional candy. But then she noticed she was finding candy wrappers more frequently in my pockets and under the bed when she cleaned. She said sugar is highly addictive. She said there was no difference between being addicted to sugar and being addicted to cigarettes. It is the same pattern of behavior. She explained the negative effects of sugar on the body. It is more dangerous than drug addiction and the addiction is hard to break. Mom said I had enough to deal with having sickle cell disease. She didn't want me to develop complications too. She had a point. Not that I liked it. But I must live with it. Sugar increases inflammation in the body. Inflammation increases complications. Eventually, I learned how important it is to control sugar intake. Now I read the labels on everything.

    My mom says the body knows when it is hungry. If we feed it nutrient-dense meals it doesn't get hungry as frequently. In my house, we eat only when we are hungry. We don't have set mealtimes. If we are not hungry in the mornings when we get up, we break our fast later in the day. There is no distinction between breakfast food, what we eat for lunch or dinner. My friends eat things like cereal or toasted pop tart. I know how to make eggs. If I want eggs for dinner, eggs it is. If I want left over dinner in the morning, that's what I eat. Sometimes I ask my mom to make pancakes for me. Sometimes mom makes French toast with almond flour. I love those. I never liked milk. But that's ok. I get plenty of calcium from the other food I eat.

Eating sprouted and fermented food has its benefits.

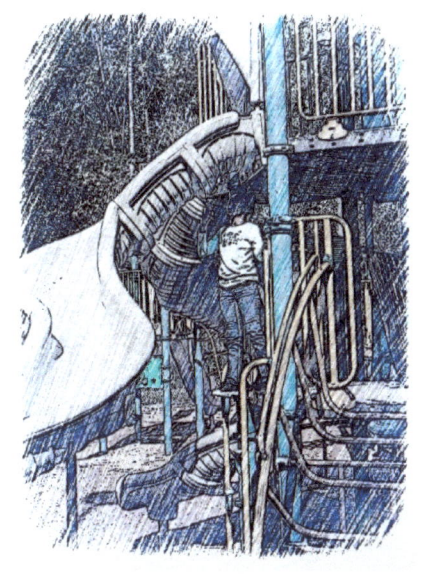

I get plenty of exercise daily. I love to dance. I go to bed dancing and wake up dancing. I can't sit still for too long. I must keep moving. My mom likes to walk. Sometimes she dances with me. We even have dance offs. I have to say, for a grown-up she has good rhythm and excellent musicality. She got that from me. What can I say? But I am a much better dancer. I do hip hop and majorette mainly. Ballet is a little too dainty for me. I don't mind jazz and contemporary. I play hard. Especially, when we go to the park. There are so many things we can do at the park. My favorite is the monkey bars. My mom says exercise is important. However, I must listen to my body. I must know when it is too much and how to pace myself. Most of all, I must stay hydrated.

I have asthma. Sometimes I must use the nebulizer. I don't like the nebulizer too much. It is noisy. When I have the dry hacking cough, it is a life saver. Mom puts some distilled water in it instead of the albuterol. The mist moistens my airways and makes me feel better. During the springtime, when my allergies are out of control, is mainly when my asthma gets active. Mom guides me through diaphragmatic breathing and pursed lips breathing. She uses eucalyptus and peppermint oil in the diffuser. I sleep with the humidifier at nights too. That helps a lot. This past spring, I had no issues with my asthma. That is a good sign. Maybe I am outgrowing it.

Why My Diet is Important.

    This is something I constantly explain to my friends. People are usually curious why I have sauerkraut, kombucha, kefir-yogurt or kimchi with my meals. Or, why my lunch doesn't look like what other kids eat. Or, why when we do eat out, I ask for water instead of juice or soda. Let me explain why this is important. There is a reason back in bible times people ate fermented food. Bacteria determine our health. I have listened to my mom give this presentation so many times that I can explain it almost as well as she does. The collection of bacteria that lives in and on the body serves to protect us from pathogens or things that cause disease. Microbial cells in the human body far outnumber human cells many times over. Basically, we are more bacteria than we are human. Our diet determines which bacteria we will have more of, helpful or harmful ones.
    When we eat unhealthy food, we feed the harmful bacteria and kill the helpful ones. The genes in the microbiome or collection of bacteria in the body outnumber the genes in the genome about 150:1. Which means the microbiome dominates and can switch the genes in the

genome on or off. This determines how your genes express themselves. Since sickle cell disease is a genetic disorder, keeping my microbiome healthy will help to control symptoms of the disease. That process is called epigenetics. While the helpful bacteria don't change the genetic code itself, they change how the genes express themselves or act. Since the food we eat mainly determines the state of our microbiome, then a healthy diet rich in pre and probiotic food will improve our body's ability to thrive and heal itself. Meaning, we will have far fewer symptoms, if any at all. The opposite is also true. If we primarily eat empty calorie processed food and especially sugar, we will signal the sickle cell genes to create more symptoms. Not only that, we will develop other complications too. Food is not the only thing that negatively impacts sickle cell disease. But it is a big part of it and one that we can completely control. Other factors affecting sickle cell are temperature and stress.

    My mom now believes the reason I was so sick all the time when I was a baby was because of the penicillin. Now, using penicillin has been beneficial and has prevented premature death in kids with sickle cell disease. It might have saved my life too. However, penicillin is an antibiotic. It does not discriminate. It kills both helpful and harmful bacteria. Babies develop their microbiome during those early years based on what they eat and are exposed to. I started taking penicillin at two weeks old. My microbiome was doomed from the start. There needs to be a balance. Since the helpful bacteria are a casualty of the penicillin, we must simultaneously replace them through our diet. However, there needs to be a window of time between when we eat probiotic rich food and when take a dose of penicillin. Otherwise, there would be no point to it.

 Mom must have been right. Once we started doing that, I started having less symptoms. I didn't need to see the doctor so often anymore and I have not been admitted to the hospital again. Everyone's experience will be different depending on the state of their microbiome. That's what makes sickle disease so hard to treat. It is highly personalized, and the treatment is more of a one size fit all. Mom thinks if there is more emphasis on wellness and eating to give our bodies the advantage, the disease would be more manageable. This is also true with the medicine. Our microbiome can help or hinder the drugs' effectiveness. Eating this way doesn't mean you never have symptoms. It simply means you have them far less frequently.

 To be honest, the first time my mother explained it to me I thought she had lost her mind. How could bacteria make me healthy? The idea that bacteria can be helpful didn't sound right. Afterall, aren't we always trying to get rid of bacteria? I fought her every step of the way. She said I had the option of going to bed hungry. Really mom?! I called her bluff and went to bed without eating one night. I refused to eat bacteria. My mom is as patient as Job and persistent as a German cockroach. Guess what was for breakfast the next morning! The same probiotic meal I didn't eat the evening before was waiting for me. There was no option B. When the hunger became too much, I ate the bacteria like I was happy to do it. It sounds a lot worse than it tastes.

    The kombucha is naturally carbonated and looks like soda. Mom made a pineapple-ginger flavored kombucha. Yum! The kefir is fermented milk. We use coconut milk. The first time I tasted it, I could think of less irritating things, like being stabbed in the eye with a rusty nail. Mom turned it into mango yogurt-kefir with a touch of vanilla. Now, that was good! My mom mixes fruits into the sauerkraut so I had a different flavor kraut each day. I prefer it like that. The kimchi is spicy. There is no redeeming that one. I like salads a lot. My mom makes them fun. She puts little chunks of cultured fruits in them. I love fries from the air fryer. I must say, my mom is right. It didn't sound at all appealing. But it makes me feel great. One day, it occurred to me that I didn't have an appetite for sweet things anymore. I asked my mom about that. She said when there is an overgrowth of fungus in our bodies, we crave sugar. These harmful fungi need sugar to thrive. When we routinely eat food rich in probiotics, we have less harmful or unhealthy bacteria, so we have less craving for sugar. Say what?!

One thing I didn't understand was why my mom and I eat different things. My mom gets sick when she eats avocado, watermelon, cantaloupe and apples. However, if she ferments them, they don't make her sick. Fermenting fruits decrease their sugar content. They are less sweet and slightly tangy. The nutritional value is much higher in cultured or fermented fruits. It is a nice balance. Seriously, my mom will ferment anything. I love apples. I can eat them all day. There are other things that she eats that I would rather take my chances at a pain crisis than eating. She drinks bone broth and eats beef liver. She even eats plain mushrooms. I have my limits. Mom says each person's microbiome is as individual as their fingerprint. No single diet will work the same for everyone. So, we each must figure what works best for our bodies and eat the food that gives our bodies the advantage to heal itself. Both mom and I took hydroxyurea. It worked for me but didn't work for her. That is weird. We are from the same family. We have the same disease. Yet our bodies need different things to stay healthy. We both love jackfruit, mangosteen, cucumber, broccoli, mangoes, berries of all kinds, greens of all kinds and star fruit, to name a few. There are so many things we can eat. Other fermented food my mom eats include tofu, tempeh, miso, kefir-cheese and coconut water kefir. I am not crazy about those either.

  Another thing my mom does is, she soaks or sprouts seeds and beans, for example, before we eat them. In addition to fermentation, these are ways to increase the nutritional value of food. We make all these at home. Food lasts longer when it is fermented. Once, my mom made a cabbage lasts 6 months by making sauerkraut with it. Sprouting seeds are inexpensive. Two tablespoons of salad mix sprouting seeds produces enough sprouts to make us both a dinner salad. So, for example, a pound of organic alfalfa seeds costs about $20 at most. We can make just over 150 cups of sprouts from that one pound of seeds. Making the coconut milk kefir usually takes about 18- 24 hours. Then she adds some prebiotics and berries and let it ferment another few hours before refrigerating it. As the probiotics in the kefir feed on the prebiotics, it thickens to a yogurt consistency. The kombucha takes the longest. It sits in the ceramic jar about 2-3 weeks. Personally, I would get it from the store. We can do that in a few minutes. But mom said it is $2.99/bottle in the store, but 19 cents/bottle when she makes it. That makes sense. That's my mom! She can squeeze six pennies from a nickel.

School Life

I am home schooled. My mom works. At first, I would meet with other homeschoolers on a ranch about 90 minutes from home two days a week. The other three days we meet at a community center. Mom felt I needed more

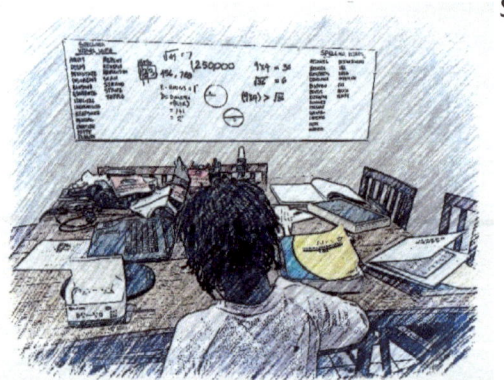

supervision and guidance than that arrangement provided. She re-arranged her work schedule to make more time to assist with my schoolwork. When mom has patients scheduled and must leave for work, I stay with my sitter. My sitter is like family. She has been my sitter for most of my life. She is strict, but a lot of fun too. It's like my mom never left. In a lot of ways, my sitter is like my grandma. When mom gets back, she sits with me to make sure I understood what I learned that day. She also looks at what else I will be doing the next day and goes through as much of it with me as she can. When we do that, I feel more prepared for my classes.

Mom likes to plan. She prepares weekly meals on Sundays. Then she portions and labels my meals for the week. She also prepares or purchase snacks and make sure I have enough water. This makes it convenient during the week. I know how to use the microwave. When I get hungry, I can simply re-heat and eat. Sometimes, I eat a salad when I want something simple and quick. All I need to do is to get a salad kit from the refrigerator and put the dressing on it.

There are benefits to being homeschooled. I love to hang out with my mom. We get to talk about life and whatever else is on my mind. We have lots of bonding time. We usually have worship together before bed. My favorite subjects are math, science and robotics. I love art too. I love to create things. I love to read. For as far back as I can remember, we have the one hour per day reading rule at home. I must read for at least an hour each day. My mom says education is important. My mom reads a lot too.

I wasn't always home schooled. My PreK year, I went to a regular school. Mom had a regular job too. But every time I got sick; mom had to take off from work. Sometimes, the school called my mom to pick me up if I started having a fever. One day, I complained to my teacher about feet hurting. She called my mom to pick me up. What I didn't tell her, was that my feet hurt because my shoes were tight. Mom warned me not to wear them anymore. They were my favorite shoes. They were Sketchers and they light up. All my friends liked them too. I didn't listen. So, mom had to take off from work to pick me up. She was not happy when she realized why my feet hurt. She gave me a stern talking to all the way home. Let me tell you about my mom's talking to. When she is mad, she could talk you into a coma. If her talking to were a prison sentence, that one would have been 25 to life.

    Mom said having to take off from work so frequently was a problem. It meant she was not reliable, through no fault of her own. She understood why her company felt the need to hire someone else. She started a business that would give her the flexibility she needed to be available whenever I needed her. She told me that may be my life someday too. I admire my mom. I started a business too. Mom said she didn't want me to think that getting a job after college was my only option. She said if I am going to spend that much money on college, I should be thinking of creating jobs instead. She always tells me life doesn't owe me a living. No one is obligated to do me any favors because I have a disease. I must work for it like anyone else. I must plan and prepare ahead. Hopefully, I can grow my business enough to pay for my own college.

The education I get at home goes beyond academics. It is also about growing up to become a productive member of society. It is about learning to navigate this life and the world we live in. It is about having appreciation and an attitude of gratitude for the opportunities we have. It is also about learning to embrace the differences in opinion and perspective of others. It is about seeing the world through the lens of another. These are things I appreciate. I admire the way my mom makes time to answer my questions. Sometimes she stops what she is doing to listen to me and assist where I need help. For me, this is priceless!

What happens when I get sick?

Thanks to God and my mom, I don't get sick very often anymore. I see the doctor annually for a well visit. I may get a cold occasionally. But they are usually short lived. There was a time I was sick and at the hospital all the time. I used to have to go to the sickle cell clinic every month. I don't like the hospital. I don't like getting shots, putting in the IV or having my blood drawn. I don't like the penicillin or hydroxyurea. I don't like albuterol or the irritating sound of the nebulizer. As much as I don't like these things, my mother loathes them. She thinks the hospital is where you go to trade your symptoms. You go in with one set of problems and leave with another or a bill you can't pay. My mom is a single parent. She must work to support us. She

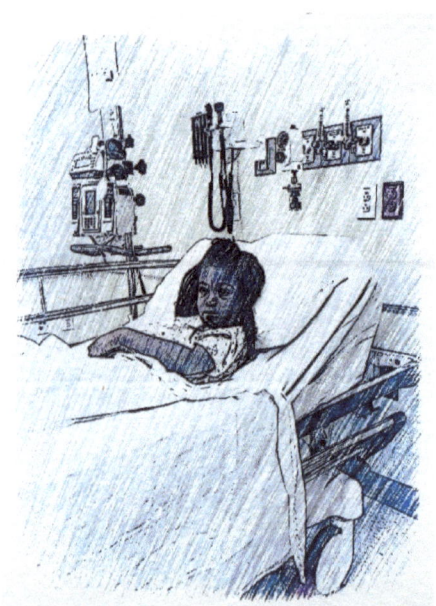

can't do that if we are in the hospital like I used to be.

My mother is a warrior. If you want her to do something, tell her it can't be done. She didn't understand why I got sick so often if I am taking the medications and keeping up with my clinic appointments. The first two years of my life were the worst. Mom has pictures of me in the hospital with tubes coming from almost every opening. Two weeks after I was born, I was put on prophylactic penicillin. I took it twice daily for 3 years. The last time I was admitted to the hospital just before turning three years old. It was bad. I used to pull out my IV. I was in a hospital bed that looked like a cage and I had restraints on. I cried all the time. I was hurting. My mother was stressed. She would pray over me all the time. Her facial expression was intense.

I ended up in the hospital that time, because I had gone to another hospital closer to home three days in a row to no avail. The first day they gave my mom Advil and albuterol and discharged me. The second day, they insist they couldn't find anything wrong with me. The third day, the nurse accused my mom of having Munchausen by proxy. They were about to discharge me again. My mom said I had been crying for a long time. She knew it wasn't my regular cry. She said I was crying, and the tears stopped flowing. My eyes were dry. We were in a room next to the nursing station. Mom said she heard one of the nurses tell another to hurry up with the discharge paperwork so they could get the screaming child out of the ER. Just about that time, mom said my body went limp and I stopped crying. She panicked and screamed for help. The nurse came rushing in she took me from my mom and yelled at the other nurse to get the doctor stat.

I had a fever of over 102 degrees. I was put on IV immediately and in the confusion, I was given an overdose of morphine. Mom said for the first time the doctor showed any interest in talking or listening to her. She gave him the number to my hematologist. I was immediately transferred to another major children's hospital. The hematologist said another couple of hours, and we could have had a different outcome. That shook my mother to the core. She said after that experience, she knew there had to be a better way. She said she felt helpless. Like she had no control over what happened. She said she sat with me in the hospital pondering what had taken place. She decided life as it was would not be sustainable. Something had to change. The one thing she knew for sure, was that would be my last hospital stay. She made sure of it.

My mom is sharp. She said she was more interested in preventing the symptoms than she was finding a cure. In her mind, it was the symptoms that kept her going back to the hospital. If she were to avoid the hospital, she would have to find a way to prevent the symptoms. She spent every waking minute she could spare researching and trying to figure what could be done. After a couple of years of trial and error, she found what works best for us. The trick was to get me to buy in. I am a strong-willed child. Mom figured all she has to do is to outlast me. She educated me as she was learning herself. It was important to her that I understood enough to make better choices on my own. I must admit, I don't always. Sometimes she has to give me a stern warning. She says I can act the fool if I want. But when I end up in the hospital, I will be going alone. Then I would straighten up. She is serious. I didn't willingly make all these dietary changes. But when I see my friends with sickle cell disease frequently in the hospital for the same complaints all the time. I knew whatever my mom is doing is more effective for us than what they are doing for themselves.

     Mom instills in me that my health is my own responsibility. She says medicine can only do so much and doctors are doing the best they can with what they have to work with. Whenever other parents would complain that what the doctor is doing isn't working for their child, mom would ask if what they, the parents, are doing is working. Because if it isn't and they keep doing the same thing they will keep getting the same outcome. Other parents often get curious about why I seem to be healthy and not have symptoms like their child. My mother tells them what she is doing differently to make that happen. There was a time I was like their child. Some responded by saying their children won't eat this or that. Or, that they don't have time for all that planning and preparation. This isn't for everyone. We all have different priorities and circumstances. We must do what works best for us.

    On the other hand, there have been a few parents who, like my mom once was, are desperate and willing to try anything. They are usually more opened to the suggestions about wellness and prevention. They have good outcomes too and are usually grateful for my mother's time and help. Another complaint is that eating healthy is too expensive. Nothing could be further from the truth. Everything in life will cost time, money or both. You must determine when and how much you are willing to pay. Admittedly, meal planning and prep take time. No matter what they pay for groceries, medical expenses and time spent in the hospital far outweigh that cost. Not only do they now have a bill they can't pay, they were not able to work during the time. Factor in the toll it takes on the body and the diminished quality of life the child experiences. Is it worth it? It wasn't for my mom and me.

All things considered; I have been blessed to have the mom I have. My mom does things for me that makes me know how loved I am. Don't get me wrong. My mom is firm and there are times she must discipline me. However, the things she does for me are priceless. My mom is a Jill of all trades and a master of many. Once, the sprinkler system busted, because the temperature fell well below zero during the night. It flooded the neighbor's yard. As you can imagine, we weren't the only ones with a busted sprinkler system. Mom tried to get a plumber to no avail. She went on YouTube and figured how to repair it herself. She went to Home Depot to get the parts she needed and repaired it in less than an hour.

One day a while ago, she was having a bad pain crisis. She managed to drive herself to the ER. My mom hates the hospital. For her to go there, the pain was bad. She was turned away without care. The doctor had reservations about prescribing narcotics for her pain. When she felt better, she had the home set up for pain management. She has a certain amount of disdain for hospital ER. She even went back to school to become a master herbalist. My mom works miracle with simple everyday herbs.

Mom developed avascular necrosis in both hips as a result of sickle cell. She did the core decompression surgery her doctor recommended. It didn't work. The pain was bad. It slowed her down. Bilateral hip replacement was her next best option. She declined. If the AVN is due to a lack of blood supply to the bone, then restoring the blood supply should fix it. Maybe the core decompression wasn't the right method for her. She figured the whole-body vibration should work to improve circulation to every part of the body. She tested her theory. She frequently used herbs she knew would improve circulation. For ten minutes every day for 5 months, she did wholebody vibration. When she had her next MRI, there was no trace of the AVN.

Let me tell you, in mom's herb cabinet, there is an herb for everything. She makes so many individual and combination of tinctures and extracts. I am glad mom thinks of everything. As she says, it is always wise to dig your well before you get thirsty. The

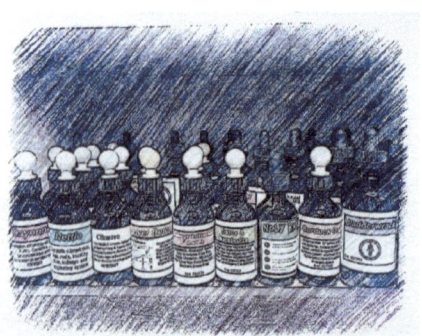

extraction takes months. Mom labels and dates each one with a description of what it can be used for. She makes salves, elixirs, lotions, soap, shampoo… You name it; mom makes it. She makes a salve with cayenne, ginger, echinacea and boswellia serrata. I use that one for regular aches and pain from hurting myself at the park. It is like magic. The elderberry syrup she makes for colds tastes better than the cold medicine from the store and works faster.

My least favorite of all the extracts is the prickly ash. I only ever had to use it once. It is a natural pain killer that also improves circulation. It stops or decrease the duration of sickle pain crisis. The whole-body vibration machine does the same thing for me. I'll use that over the prickly ash any day. Mom has a lot of tools in her toolbox to keep us healthy. We drink a lot of herbal teas. Mom makes some terrific combinations of herbal teas. One of my favorites has cinnamon, apple, hibiscus, lemon, ginger, chamomile and stevia herb. It reminds me of apple pie. And by the way, remember that overgrowth of fungus I mentioned earlier? The pau d'arco and olive leaf tea we drink takes care of that too. I have to say, I am glad we don't often get sick. But when we do, we can take care of it at home. As mom says, wellness is our plan

A and the doctor is our plan B. When I grow up, I want to be just like my mom!

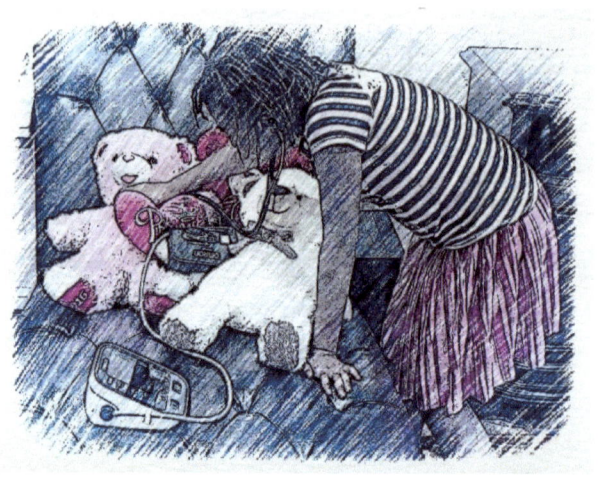

My Dreams and Fears

My greatest aspiration is to create a wellness protocol for improving quality of life for all children living with sickle cell disease. My mom said the medical treatment protocol right now is a work in progress. The quest for a universal cure remains elusive. Each person presents with a different cluster of symptoms. I don't have all the answers. Mom and I talk about this all the time. She thinks the conversation between doctor and patient needs to be different. Doctors can only work with what they see. They must work within their scope of practice. Parents have a responsibility too to pursue wellness to complement what the doctors are doing. When it comes to treating the disease, we miss the forest for the tree, as mom puts it. We look at the effect of the disease on the body without simultaneously focusing on the effect of the state of the body on the disease. Mom thinks that is the missing link. That is where those living with the disease need to pay most attention. The doctors are already doing their part. We need to do ours.

It appears to me that both are relevant. We will always need doctors to treat the acute symptoms of sickle cell disease. Mom thinks they do a good job with the capabilities they currently have. Medicine has come a long way in treating this disease. There are sickle cell clinics all over the world working hard to improve the lives of those living with the disease. They have had a measure of success. Much has been addresses about sickle cell awareness. However, the medical aspect is where the emphasis is placed. Wellness is the critical missing element, as my family has discovered and live by. I am a third-generation person with the disease in my family. My grandma is still alive and doing well. My mom and I do relatively well. My aunt does well too. My mom has been the maverick in the family. Her emphasis is always on what we need to do to contribute to our own well-being. Wellness is a way of life for us.

    I do not believe that we are unique. There have been other families living with the disease who find what works for them and thrive. Some have inquired of my mom about pursuing wellness for their child with the disease. Mom usually start off by saying, if they are looking for a quick solution or have acute symptoms, they need to see their doctors about that. However, if they are looking to improve their health and willing to invest the time and effort, she educates them on pursuing wellness. Wellness is not a quick fix. It is a journey. There isn't a formula that will work the same way for everyone. It is individualized. It requires us to be proactive. Based on our experience, improving the microbiome has been the most beneficial approach. Food became our medicine.

    Usually, when families experience the positive effect of pursuing wellness, they are sold on the concept of wellness to better manage the disease. Mom re-emphasizes it takes time, so they need to be patient and stay the course. Families have reported drastic changes over periods as short three months. While some families reported periods of up to a year to achieve the results they were looking for. One mother, whose child was severely affected by the disease, had been on frequent transfusions with iron overload as a side effect. She was so grateful when one year later was told her son was doing so well, he no longer needed the transfusions. His risk of having a stroke had significantly diminished. Before pursuing wellness, she stated the doctor told her there was no avoiding the transfusions given her son's risk for a stroke and that they simply had to treat the iron overload that came with it. Another parent decided to make wellness a priority for the family. Within three months, not only had their son been pain free, but the entire family's health and well-being improved. There are countless other examples. The takeaway, for me, is that when wellness is the journey; good health is the destination.

    I am just a kid. There is a lot I don't know and things I can't do yet. Mom said if I feel strongly about wanting to help other kids like myself, I can start by sharing my experience in a book. Children all over the world can read and benefit from my experience. That I can do. But I will need some help. I am glad she said a book. Secretly, I am shy. I couldn't do presentations and public speaking like my mom. I get performance anxiety. I mean anxiety so bad; it feels like my heart would stop. Let me tell you about my first piano recital…

    On the day of the recital, I did everything I could to stall. I was having a visceral reaction to the thought of playing in front of a crowd. My mom said I had to go. She just didn't get it. I am not brave like she is. It is usually a 30-minute drive to the recital location. That day, it felt like five minutes only. My mom pulled up to the building. My palms were sweaty. I could hardly breathe. I could feel every heartbeat vibrating in my chest. As I entered the building, my knees shook about 7.5 on the Richter. It felt like I needed fresh underwear. My mom walked up to me, placed her arm around my shoulder and told me everything will be fine. I just wanted it to be over!

My name was 5th on the list. I don't think I heard any of the kids before me. I was too busy trying to calm myself. My name was about to be called. It was do or die. I took a deep breath. I picked up my folder. Put my shoulders back. Held my head high and walked up like I owned that stage. I was about to fake it until I could make it. I made it through that night, and I was proud of my performance. But I still dread having to do anything like that. It is stressful. Mom said she was like me when she was a kid. She used to have performance anxiety too. I cannot imagine my mother ever being like this. Maybe there is hope for me, after all!

When I grow up

I don't know yet what I want to do when I grow up. I can be anything I want to be. I have plenty of time to think about that. I am only 8. I will keep growing my e-commerce business. I will write a series of books. I want to do something I enjoy. The one thing I am positive about is that I would love to promote wellness and prevention as the main way of attaining optimal health. I think it is better to avoid becoming sick in the first place. My experience living with sickle cell disease has taught me a lot about life and living. They are not the same.

I dream of a time when all children living with the disease will know what it is to truly live… to have a good quality of life… to not experience pain… There was a time when growing up was an optimistic thought for children with this disease. Today, we are living longer. But we are not necessarily having a better quality of life. Many are merely surviving. It is that elusive good quality of life that fascinates me. My life is not perfect. Under the circumstances, I can't complain. I have far more good than bad days. Sure, I have some limitations. But I enjoy my life. I would love each child to experience what I experience plus more. To discover what works best for them and to explore every available option to thrive despite the disease.

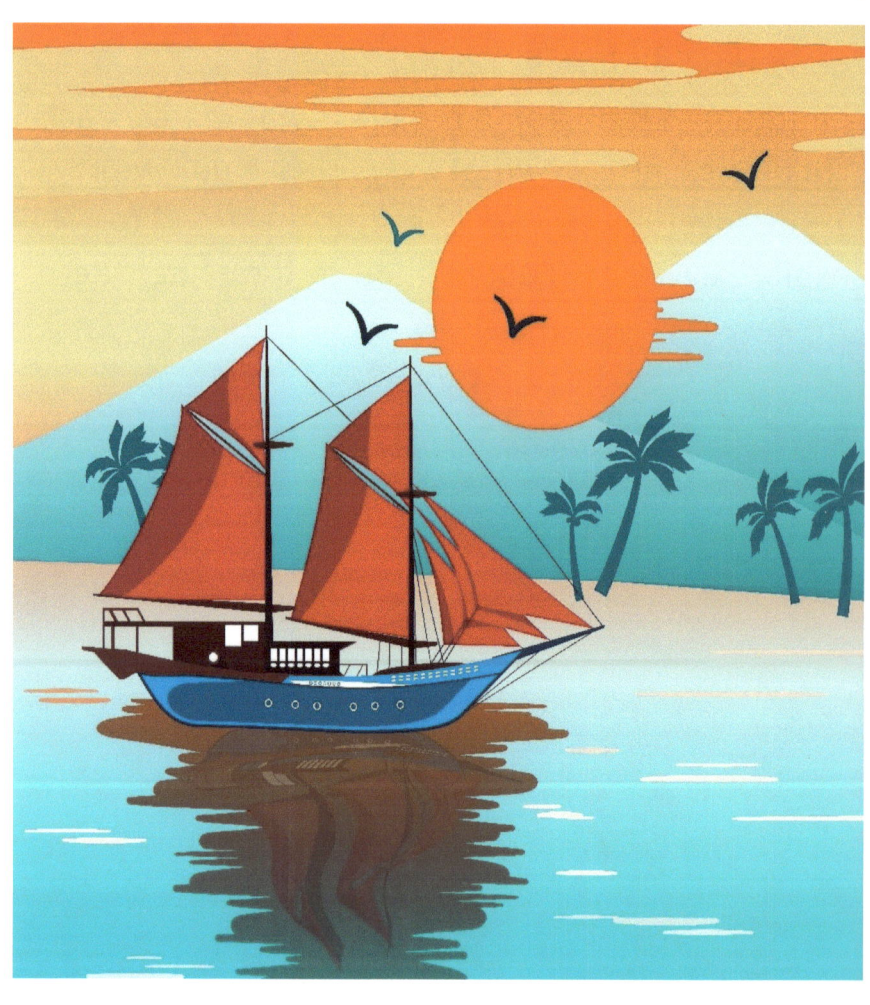

I couldn't change the direction of the wind. So I adjusted my sail and kept on my journey.

www.ingramcontent.com/pod-product-compliance
Lightning Source LLC
Chambersburg PA
CBHW042218050426
42453CB00001BA/6